I0100384

CALM

BEFORE THE SCAN

CALM

BEFORE THE SCAN

How To Stop Worrying About
Cancer Recurrence

JOE BAKHMOUTSKI

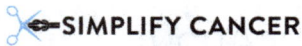

✂ SIMPLIFY CANCER

http://simplifycancer.com

ISBN   978-0-6485995-4-8 (print)
           978-0-6485995-5-5 (ebook)

Editor: Ine Baerdemaeker
Cover design: Boris Sabranovic
Interior design: Adina Cucicov

First Edition

Disclaimer: This book is not intended as a substitute for the medical advice of physicians.

Please note: Some names in this book have been changed to preserve the privacy of individuals.

CONTENTS

THE FEAR ALL CANCER SURVIVORS SHARE

The fear of cancer recurrence, as it is affectionately known in the world of psycho-oncology, affects as much as 87 percent of those who have had cancer. You might know this fear as *scanxiety*, which some patients call it.

Or you might not have a name for it at all. It doesn't matter, since you are intimately familiar with the gut-churning feeling you get from the excruciating uncertainty you face every time you go for a scan, or see your specialist to find out whether the cancer is back. This fear robs you of your freedom to look ahead and make plans, filling your head with worry, confusion, and doubt. It drains you of the mental energy you need to be creative, dragging you away from the precious time you have with your loved ones, your friends, and your life's work.

My Little Epiphany

I remember how this worry welled up inside me two weeks before my first yearly check-up. It started with a reminder in my calendar, which caused an avalanche of questions to enter my mind: *I wonder how it will go this time? Will my oncologist get the results in time? How accurate are they anyway? Will I find out for sure?*

This niggling back pain I've been having—is it cancer? Wait, is it growing, has it spread? And if it is, is there more chemo, or another surgery, or is this it, and nothing more can be done?

The worries kept buzzing around in my mind, taking me deeper, and deeper, down the spiral of doom. Nothing made sense. I could not hold a conversation or make plans because at the back of my mind, a little voice kept asking, over and over again: *What if the cancer is back? What if it's back? What if it has come back?*

There was no answer, and the more I tried to put those thoughts away, the more they came back to haunt me. It didn't matter if I was in the shower, on my way to work, or hanging out with a friend—I could not stop thinking about it.

Can they tell that I'm exploding on the inside? Can I hold it in without losing it completely?

One day, I could not take it anymore. I had to get out of the house, try and clear my head. It was already late. I closed the gates behind me and crossed the street, making my way to the path running along the train tracks.

It was pitch dark, and I could only see a few steps ahead of me. I cursed and howled into the night, furious at the injustice of it all.

I kept asking myself, *What is it, what is something that I can do about the whole cancer thing coming back?*

The answer was always the same. *Well, nothing, it's not up to me. It's all biology and random chance.*

But if I couldn't do anything about cancer coming back, then what about the rest of my life—did I have that under control?

I stopped in my tracks and looked up. The moon was peeking out between the dark clouds above, a tiny shape filled with light.

I asked myself, "Am I living my best life right now?"

Immediately, without having a clue of what my best might look like, I knew I was not where I wanted to be.

Because if I was living my best life, doing the best I could do, on my terms, then I could live with the worry about cancer coming back, I could deal with uncertainty because it's only one part of me, something I can manage.

The only thing that mattered was whether I was at my absolute best, for if the cancer had returned, then I could deal with whatever came my way. I wouldn't have any regrets about the life I'd been living, and I wouldn't be able to fault myself in any way.

How can you explain something that you can't put into words just yet?

The life I had on that day was another chance I had been given, and in many ways, I was letting it go to waste.

Feeling sorry for myself for getting cancer and putting my family through the difficulties that come with cancer treatment, I had never considered the possibility of having a good life after cancer.

While I couldn't control what the cancer might do, nobody could stop me from getting my life in order. I had the power to make sure any worries I might have about cancer did not control my life in any way.

All this time, I'd been looking for things that could go wrong, so wasn't it time to look for opportunities to make things right?

How This Guide Will Help You

In this guide, I share the four key elements you need to take down your worry about cancer coming back, and to bring more energy, fulfillment, and fun into your life after cancer.

This simple framework is built around the letters of the word SCAN. It is based on my experiences, working with hundreds of people who strive to move away from anxiety towards a more calm, measured, and impactful life beyond cancer.

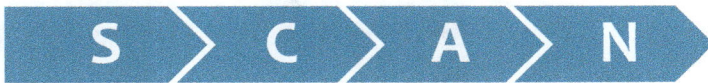

The four key elements to SCAN your life for what you can make right are:

Support—building a deeper connection with the people you care about the most

Contribute—making a difference that is consistent to you and your values

Appreciate—finding peace with yourself and your own place in the world

Negotiate—working around life's inevitable changes and challenges

In the next four chapters, I will break down each element of the SCAN framework in a way that you can apply to your life. This will help you deal with your fear of cancer coming back.

PART 1

SUPPORT
FOR YOURSELF AND FOR THOSE YOU CARE ABOUT THE MOST

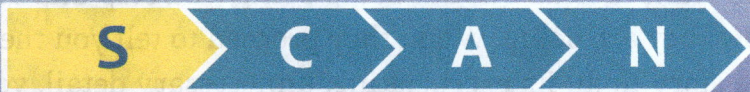

S **C** **A** **N**

We are not meant to suffer through our struggle alone. This is the reason we make friends. It's why we fall in love. It is what compels us to build cities, join clubs, and find shelter in our communities. We want to know that our people will be there to back us when the going gets rough.

The first few days I spent in the hospital went by in a blur, but once I'd settled into the chemo routine, the days grew long and I started feeling lonely on my own. So when my best friend said she and her partner would drop by after work, I got excited to have some company.

After walking in and greeting me, she looked me over as if I was a new dress in a shop window, "You do look good."

"You almost sound disappointed," I said.

"No, it's just that I expected... Never mind, good to see that you are well looked after in here. So how's it all going?"

You know how it can be a little awkward when you bump into someone you haven't seen in a while, like a former colleague or someone you went to school with ages ago? You want to head off, but being polite, you stop and ask how they are doing. When they proceed to tell you their life story in all its excruciating, unnecessary detail, you stand there, nodding your head, hoping something comes up to distract them so you can make a run for it.

This time, I was the one telling my life story. When I ran out of air, I stopped mid-sentence. My friend did not seem to notice, as she peered out the window. "That's not a bad view, actually. Well, I suppose we'd better leave you to it… Remember, we're only a phone call away. If there's anything I can do to help, let me know."

I didn't know it then, but my wife had texted a few of my closest friends saying I'd appreciate a visit. That knowledge might have made this visit more bearable and filled me with humiliation for having them goaded into dropping by to see me.

Instead, I fell into a vast, suffocating emptiness. I stared at the fading world on the opposite side of the window, hoping that one day, there would be more people out there waiting for me.

This is one of the side effects of cancer—it presents our personal relationships in a new light. You look at your friend or workmate in a particular way, and it can take a big shake-up like cancer to reveal how close or how far apart you may be right now. It can often go in unexpected directions. People you might not have been close with can step up and be there for you in a significant way.

There are many ways to support someone in a difficult time, but it starts and ends with the feeling. Whether you are going through a difficult time, or you are there for someone who is facing struggle, both of you are looking for an emotional experience that is aligned with your values. For it is not the act that matters, or the resources that go into it, whether it's time, money, or energy, but the emotional charge that you both receive in return. If the person receiving the support feels understood, and the person supporting them feels appreciated, everybody wins.

It can be tricky to figure out what help you might be looking for yourself at the best of times, and it is that much harder to find out what someone else is looking for in their moment need. Even when you know them as well as you think you do, what they are looking for might change depending on the moment you find them in.

Going with your gut can be a lifesaver, but having structure around it can give you a tremendous advantage. Not only will your loved one or friend look to you as a source of calm and understanding, but you are also likely to feel more appreciated and cherished because of the difference you are making for someone on their terms.

You cannot give help without accepting it in return. It goes both ways—for if you cannot find a way to talk about what's troubling you, then how can you pick up on the distress signals others might be sending your way? And if you cannot find a way to tell someone how they can support you in a meaningful way, then how will you know that the help you are giving them is what they actually wanted in the first place?

Giving help and accepting help from others does not need to happen at the same time, but you want to be in a position where you are ready to give help, just as you can gracefully accept help in turn. Support is not a trade-off, but an acknowledgement that everything in life goes both ways and that our relationships are filled with meaning and purpose.

Support is a life raft that is out on the storming sea. To keep the balance, you draw people in and help them recognise their own struggle. You do that when you listen. When there is no judgement or advice, and you feel truly heard, you are free to explore the edges of your struggle and make sense of it as you talk about it. Making sense of their own experience is an incredible gift you can give someone going through a difficult time.

To hold the balance when you are living the struggle, it's crucial to acknowledge that people in your life need guidance. No matter how well they know you, they will never guess what type of support you are looking for at any given moment. If they care about you, they will want you to guide them. To get your people behind you on your terms, it's crucial for you to direct them to meaningful action. This will also prevent them from providing help that you don't want because you are direct and explicit about the support you need.

These are the two forces that we look to for balance over time:

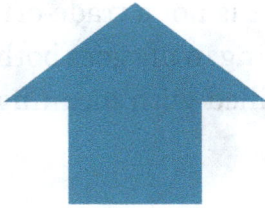

LISTEN

• You will draw people in to become the source of calm and understanding

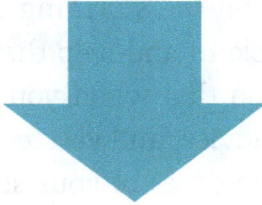

DIRECT

• Your people will be grateful to support you on your terms when you direct them to help you in a meaningful way

Make It Easy for People to Help You

When you are in trouble, most people around you want to help, but they don't know how. Often, they don't want to risk offending you in any way. It's only natural—they don't want to say the wrong thing that might make you feel worse, only for them to feel stupid and insensitive in the end.

In order for you to have the support you want in your life, it's vital to guide your people towards helping you in a meaningful way. This does not mean you will ask them to do something complicated or grand, only that you tell them what you would appreciate in some way. You might think that telling people what you expect them to do is pushy or even rude, but those who truly care about you will be grateful that you make it easy for them to support you.

Proper support has to be a great FIT for you and those around you:

Frank—You might hold back your troubles when you don't want to be a burden, but bringing your worries out into the open helps people understand what you are going through. Not only does it help them come to terms with what is troubling you, but it also saves you the hassle of finding the right thing to say or keeping it from boiling up from within. It can be incredibly helpful to you and those you care about when you bring up your worries and concerns about cancer coming back as part of the conversation you are already having.

Informed—It can be tough to make sense of the challenges that surround you, much less explain them to someone else. When we feel lost, it often helps to zero in on the facts. For example, when you are worried about cancer coming back, it can help to ask your specialist about your chances of recurrence and what the options are if it happens. It enables you to direct your own attention and the attention of those who care about you towards the reality of the situation rather than the uncertainty around it.

Timely—Your circumstances can often change, and so does the way you feel. Some days, you might want some time alone with your thoughts, and on another day, you want to be with your family or talk to your friend. It's natural to not only want different things, but also to express your feelings in such a way that they cannot be misinterpreted or misunderstood.

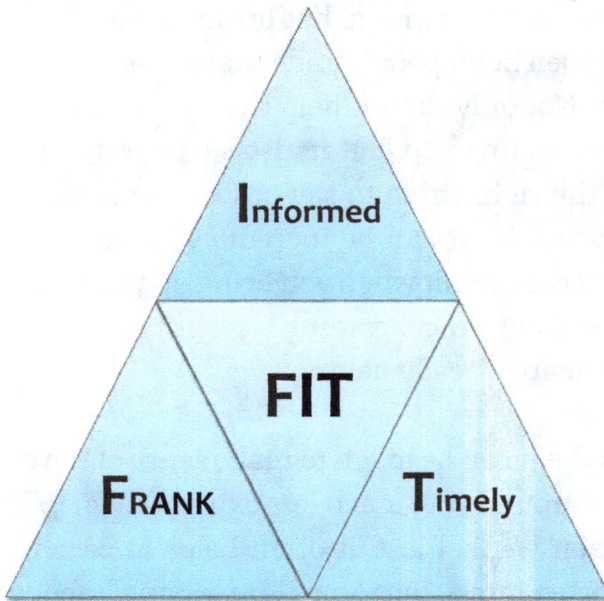

When you obsess about finding the best way to share your thoughts and express your feelings in a way that others expect from you, that takes away the precious energy you need to enjoy the time you pznd together. It's much easier to be frank and direct about what you are experiencing so that there is no guesswork or misunderstanding involved. It also means people can't feel angry or upset, since you are giving them an insight in your emotions. Speaking your mind can take a little used to, but it can free you from overanalysing, or worse, misjudging situations.

Exercise: Direct your people into action

This exercise will help you get in touch with the type of support you are looking for. It will show you how to direct your people towards meaningful action without feeling awkward or misunderstood.

Taking a few minutes to write down your answers can reveal new details that you have never considered or thoughts that have never occurred to you in the rush of daily life.

What might be the situation in your life that you find hard to deal with?

If your partner/friend/workmate could read your mind, what would be the obvious thing they do for you?

If they knew exactly what you wanted, what would they avoid doing at any cost?

How can you direct your partner/friend/workmates towards meaningful action in a way that will leave no room for misunderstanding?

My personal choice would be to send out an email that outlines all the ways people around me can help. This can be a list of tasks or activities that are currently challenging for you or ways to keep you company. Here is an example:

Hi guys,

As you might know, I just finished my cancer treatment and I'm not feeling my best. It'd be great to hang out if you have time on weeknights or the weekend. Also, we would appreciate help with any of the following:

- *Driving me to and from doctor's appointments*
- *Doing groceries*
- *Babysitting*

If you ever have time for any of the above, reply to this email and let me know.

Joe

Don't wait for others to guess how they can help you in a difficult time. Instead, direct them to meaningful action. Being clear and specific helps to define your expectations for people around you and makes it easier for them to pick and choose, so they can support you in a way that is comfortable for them. If they care about you, they will be grateful for the opportunity to support you on your terms.

Listen to Ease the Pain

Do you remember a time when you sat down with your partner or a friend, and they were completely absorbed in the conversation, hanging on to your every word? They asked deep, thoughtful questions, and the words flowed like a river. You never felt rushed, and there was nowhere you'd rather be, as if you were enjoying a patch of cool shade on a hot summer's day.

This happened to me when an old friend came to visit me at the hospital during chemo. The world was crumbling all around me, and she came to be by my side and listen. It was such a relief to be heard, and nothing else mattered. There was no need to put on a brave face because I wasn't judged on my performance, and I could speak my mind freely.

And it felt right to be myself, to be honest and direct, without any drama or show, to bask in full and undivided attention, and to drive the worry away from the inside.

When was the last time this happened to you? For many of us, a conversation like this is a luxury that does not happen often enough. Often, it's the opposite—you run across someone for whom listening equals waiting for you to stop talking so that they can barge in with their own agenda.

It is only when you feel truly heard and appreciated that you come alive. When you are recognised for your authentic, true self, any doubt or hesitation falls away, and because of that, you are ready to listen back.

For your message to carry, people need to feel that you care. Before they put their trust in you and your ideas, people want to be heard. If you want to get their attention, you have to give them your attention first.

✎ Exercise: Listening for support

People's needs and wants fluctuate depending on how they feel and what is going on around them. To eliminate any misunderstanding or guesswork, be direct and ask your friend, partner, or colleague who might be struggling right now:

What's the one thing I can do for you today?

If they don't tell you, ask about a different timeframe:

What's the one thing that I can do for you next week?

If you believe there is something you can do to support them, it helps to be specific and make it easy for them to say either yes or no:

Can I come over and visit?

Can I drive you to the hospital?

Can I help with babysitting/groceries/school drop-offs?

If you are not ready to commit to anything, then you don't need to offer help. It does not make you a bad person, but someone who knows their boundaries. It is much better to offer no help at all than to give half-hearted promises. On the other hand, you can still let the other person know you care.

As you listen, you help the other release their tension and worry by making sense of their experience, and by doing so, you become the person they turn to for calm and understanding.

When you listen, you give validation to their experience. You pull people towards you because their feelings are recognised, and they feel validated in their experience.

Being a good listener is a rare and precious gift that you can give to the people you care about. It is also an opportunity to be present in the moment, and reflect on where you are in life and the bond you may share.

While it may not always be easy to commit your time, money, or energy, giving help can be simple once you know what people want. You don't have to worry about sidelining them or second-guessing yourself, because you are giving them a chance to express their true feelings and share what they are looking for now.

You might not currently be in a place where you are ready to offer help, and that's okay. We go through difficult periods at times where we need to sort out the situation at hand before we can do the same for others. Still, you want to let your friend or workmate know what you can and cannot do for them, or else you might lead them to believe that you don't care. If I had the chance to go back in time to a similar situation, I would say this: "I'm sorry you have to go through this, and I wish could do more than talking to you about it the way we do now, but there are some things I must resolve for my family before I can step up and be there for you."

In the push/pull model of support, you are ready to help those around you when they need it the most, and you are compelled to accept help in return. Similarly to love and respect, the support that exists in your life needs to be mutual. When it comes to supporting someone in a difficult time, it is the experience that counts, not the act. What you do is easily forgotten, but the feeling both parties get from it will last. Just as the photo from the family trip you took as a kid can stir up feelings that you may have long forgotten, so does the memory of a kind word. A moment you shared with someone in a difficult time can bring you closer together and bring more of those good vibes into your life.

PART 2

TAKE AWAY
WORRY THROUGH
CONTRIBUTION

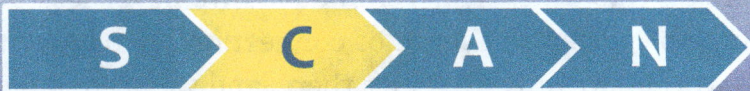

S C A N

After you were diagnosed with cancer and went through remission, did you feel like going back to the life you had before was just not the same anymore? Maybe you don't fit in, and some of those things you enjoyed so much seem trivial now, like you're just going through the motions? Even the plans you had for the future may now feel pointless and ordinary, almost banal.

It is a very natural situation when your life has been impacted in a dramatic way, which is what happens when you go through cancer. If there was no shift in how we think, feel, or look at the world and how we fit in, then we would stop responding and be stuck in some cosmic version of Groundhog Day forever.

When you feel like you have lost something, it's merely a reminder that you need to find it again. I often think back to my childhood, when my grandma would search all over the house for her glasses. She would raise her hands in frustration, "I have searched high and low for those glasses, but it's like they have vanished." I pointed at her brow, "But grandma, they are right there, on your forehead!" She only smiled, "Just to think they've been there all this time." This reminds me we never lose our source of power, the sense of connection we have with the world—we only forget it's there, and we need to pick it up again.

Your cancer experience has expanded the way you look at the world, and even the way you see yourself. Your perspective has changed, and so must your way of living. To get those elements in line, you want to invest in new experiences that will pull worry aside and help you lead a happier, more fulfilled life.

Devote Yourself to a Cause You Can Control

In the infinite world of possibilities that surround us today, there are many worthy causes you can turn to. Some of these may already be a part of your life in some way; others you may have considered, but never had the opportunity to explore. The cause that you turn to does not need to become your crowning achievement or some holy grail, but it does need to hit home for you. You have the power to choose projects, set goals, and be around people that are in line with the person you are today. Investing your time and energy in a cause that you believe in will make you feel that, once again, you belong.

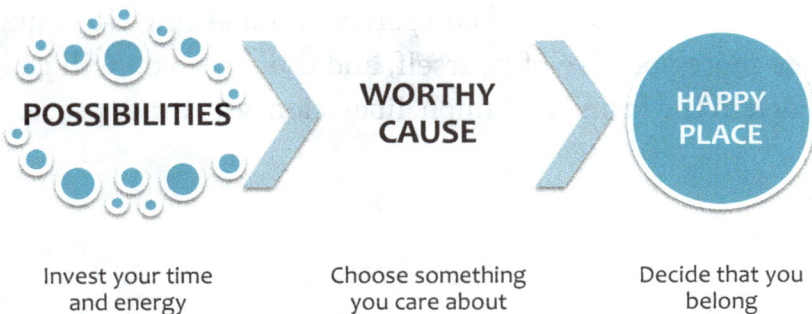

POSSIBILITIES > **WORTHY CAUSE** > **HAPPY PLACE**

Invest your time and energy

Choose something you care about

Decide that you belong

Being a part of something beyond yourself, be it your own project or a cause you choose to be part of, can pull you away from worry. Devoting yourself to things you can control or influence in some way will give you a new way of living that is more exciting, more fun, more YOU!

This does not take away from the difference that you are already making today, be it with the people you care about or your life's work. When you conspire to make a greater difference, you learn more about yourself and what you are capable of.

You don't need to drop things you can't live without. You don't have to pick and choose in how you divvy up your time and energy. It's the natural process of evolution where new habits replace old ones, and new activities replace those that may not be serving you any longer.

It's All About YOU

Helping others helps you in direct proportion to how much you care. The more real and personal something is to you, the more you give of yourself, and the more you will get back in the form of triumph, liberation, and inner peace.

This is how you can build the contribution around YOU:

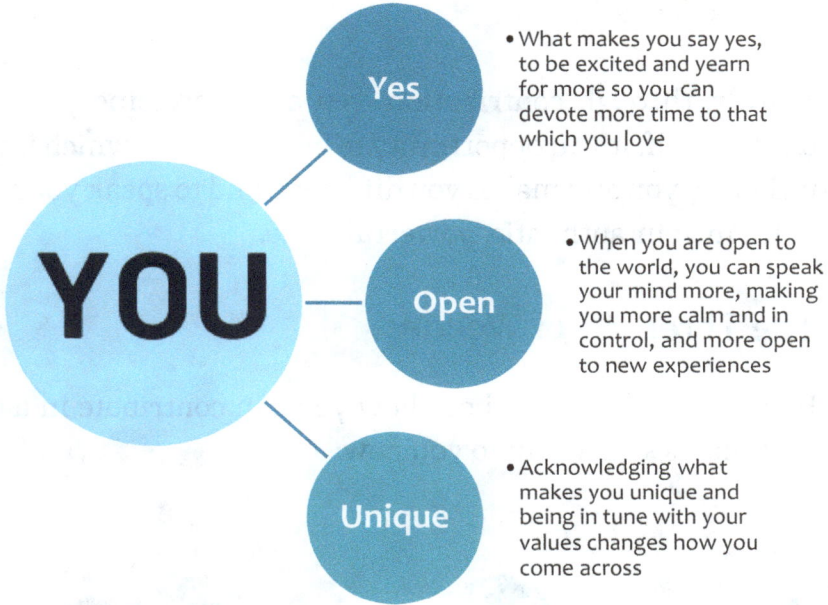

Yes
- What makes you say yes, to be excited and yearn for more so you can devote more time to that which you love

YOU

Open
- When you are open to the world, you can speak your mind more, making you more calm and in control, and more open to new experiences

Unique
- Acknowledging what makes you unique and being in tune with your values changes how you come across

First of all, the idea or event should be something you want to say "Yes!" to without even thinking about it twice. It's exciting because it's an opportunity to try something you've never done before, to take a big, bold step forward or meet new, interesting people.

Secondly, when you make a difference in a way that is true to yourself and your way of life today, you open yourself up to new possibilities and experiences that help you grow. You are more open to receiving the recognition and support you deserve, and you have greater control of what is going on around you, which helps you keep your worries in check.

Thirdly, through contribution, you are expressing your one true self. It's an opportunity to bring out that which is unique to you and makes you different, and to speak your truth in your authentic, powerful voice.

The Three Ws of Wonder

Here is one way to find out how you can contribute in a way that is significant to you now:

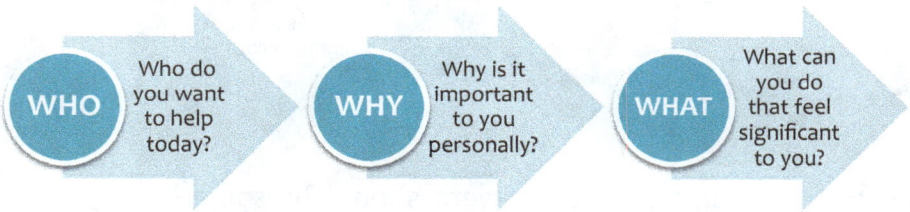

WHO Who do you want to help today? **WHY** Why is it important to you personally? **WHAT** What can you do that feel significant to you?

Exercise: Identify who you want to serve, and how

These questions can help you clarify your purpose so that you can stay on track towards your dreams despite the challenges that will stand in your way.

Who is the person that looks up to you the most right now?

_____

Who has lived through a similar struggle that needs help right now?

_____

_____

Do you feel that helping them is something you must do, and why?

_____

_____

If you could do one thing this year to make a difference in a way that is significant to you and your values, it would be to...

_____

_____

When you give your best to those in your life that you care about the most, when you devote your creativity towards meaningful projects that help your community, when you give a helping hand to those who may be struggling right now, when you get behind a cause that speaks to you on a deep, personal level, you push worry out of your way.

It may not be easy to start, but you have lived through your cancer, and you are still here. You have the strength to give your best and contribute in a way that is consistent with who you are today and how you want to see yourself in the future.

PART 3

APPRECIATE
THAT WHICH WAS
(ALMOST) TAKEN AWAY

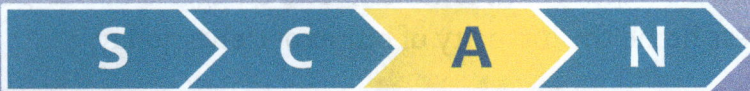

S · C · A · N

Just before starting chemo, I found myself with my pants down, naked in a locked chamber. Sitting on a raised chair, as if on a throne wrapped in plastic, I held my proud male organ in my left hand. In my right—a small plastic jar with a yellow cap. The thought of my frozen sperm as a safety net for the future was a small comfort. My oncologist was right, of course, we might want a second kid—that is, if I ever made it past the cancer treatment.

My eyes moved slowly from the uninspired cover of the one and only porn movie to the stained carpet below. Clearly, this room had not been designed with the customer experience in mind. Still, I decided to put my imagination to good use and do what must be done.

Three years later, I was walking on the lush, green lawn in the botanical gardens, not even a ten-minute walk from our house. Max was running up ahead, with his sideways shuffles. He was constantly one step away from tripping over, but that did not temper his enthusiasm one little bit. "Flaaah!", he was screaming with excitement, pointing to the field of wildflowers up ahead. I couldn't help but grin and wonder—*Is this real? Can I keep living this dream, and there is no going back to cancer?* The struggles of our past press home the intensity of our experience today.

After surviving cancer, you are constantly waiting for something to happen. Caught between the all clear and the all out disaster, you lose your ability to dream, aim high, and break rules.

Now, more than ever, you need to bring back your sense of wonder, possibility, and exploration so you can come to terms with uncertainty. As children, we look at the world with wonder, and we embrace the fact that we don't know things for certain because we know we can stumble on something extraordinary and have fun with it.

Rediscovering Your Sense of Wonder

Rediscovering our sense of wonder begins by making sense of what went wrong, the past hurts that we inadvertently hold onto, and those plans that did not turn out as expected. The confusion and mixed feelings keep piling up, tripping over each other, and we can only serve ourselves better when we make headway with untangling our past, present, and the future.

Our aim is to keep our past from spilling over into the present, and to prevent the worries of today from clouding over the future.

PAST

- Past is behind you
- Opportunity to learn and reflect
- Highlight what you like, and move on

WONDER

FUTURE

- Your Line of Control
- Everything is possible
- Nothing to lose, and everything to gain
- It's a dream that begins today

PRESENT

- Second chance at life
- This moment matters
- You have so much to give!
- Give before you get

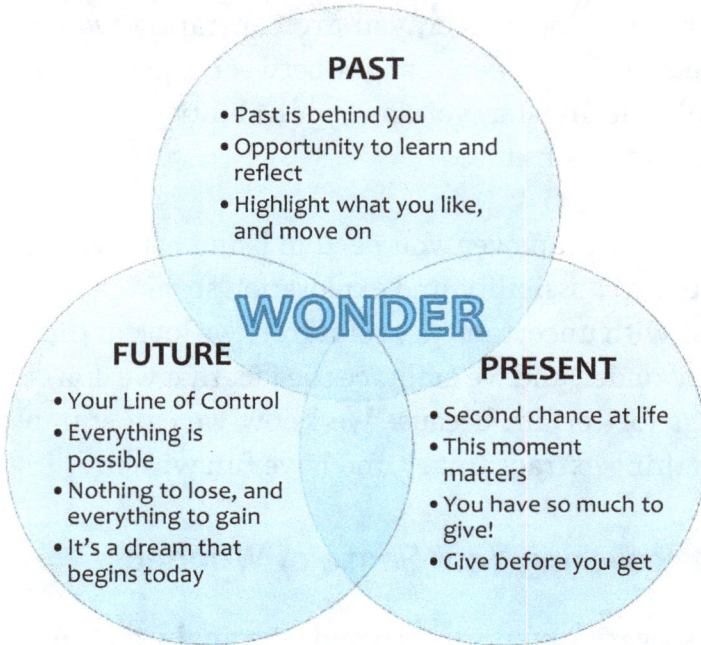

Exercise: Untangling past, present, and future

Let's sort through situations that bring back bad memories, make life difficult today, or cast clouds over the future. We will do this without rationalising them as they appear today or questioning why they happened in the first place.

We want to classify those times and situations in a way that is looking to the future from the perspective of what you can turn around if you really put your mind to it, or if you decide that there is nothing to be done to change the situation in any way.

Write out the key situations that have made your life difficult:

Cannot be undone	Can be turned around

Let's look at the situations you listed above to decide whether these are experiences that you would like to hold on to (in the sense that you want to target your efforts) and immerse yourself in, or perhaps let this experience go (in the sense that it is not affecting your daily life in a significant way).

You may need to split up your experience into distinct parts—when it comes to cancer, for example, you can-not change your diagnosis or the necessity of treatment, but you can influence how you deal with pain, or how you tackle your worry about cancer coming back.

Now, put a tick next to the situations that you want to hold on to, and a cross next to the ones you would like to let go.

You will notice that some of those events are complex and may have been affecting your life for a significant period of time. We cannot shove them aside at a moment's notice, but we can begin the process of looking at life's challenges in a way that looks towards the future, where we can direct our efforts to that which we can control.

A Daily Appreciation Ritual

If I am honest with myself and with you, I often fall into the trap of everyday life, when a myriad of things are demanding my attention. I forget where I came from and start taking beautiful, precious things for granted. The simple beauty of holding my younger son's hand as he learns how to walk. The blissful pleasure of sitting out on the deck, as the morning sun comes out to play. The gift of my older boy giving me a high five before he runs on through the school gates. There are times I forget that all this was nearly taken away, and that appreciating the life I have been given is not a choice, but a virtue, a sacred duty that I must uphold each and every day.

When you elevate appreciation from a fleeting, impromptu thought to a daily ritual, your cancer will not hold sway over you any longer. It merely exists as a memory, while the present, all-consuming and powerful, takes it place.

Appreciating the people and circumstances we find our-selves in is vital, but gratitude begins with yourself, in recognising your way of life and how far you have come. Appreciation is the way we ground ourselves in our experience:

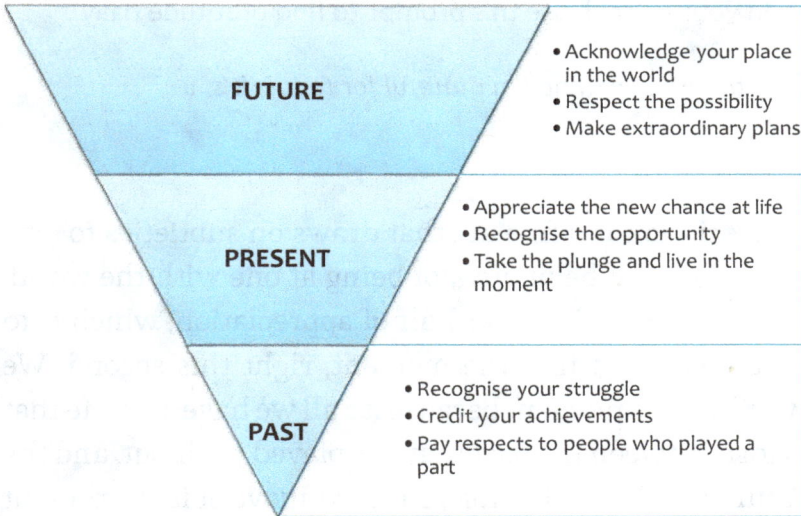

FUTURE
- Acknowledge your place in the world
- Respect the possibility
- Make extraordinary plans

PRESENT
- Appreciate the new chance at life
- Recognise the opportunity
- Take the plunge and live in the moment

PAST
- Recognise your struggle
- Credit your achievements
- Pay respects to people who played a part

You want to celebrate life in all its imperfections, with the changes and challenges it brings, because it's a part of who you are. Isn't it true that life wasn't easy before cancer? Isn't it true you had to overcome setbacks and live through challenging times that disoriented and numbed you at times?

Your struggles can bring out a new appreciation for yourself, and your place in the world, but only if you let them.

When you cultivate appreciation, and let it grow, it will add more joy and fulfilment to your daily life.

> ### ✐ Exercise: One-minute gratitude detector
>
> In your journal, use this prompt to find gratitude daily:
>
> *If there's one thing I'm grateful for today, it's...*

Appreciation is a fine art that draws on subtleties to give you a sense of belonging, of being at one with the world. This speaks to the other half of appreciation, which is to throw yourself into the moment, right this second. We worship this moment because it's all we have: in a life that is torn between the past that has played itself out, and the future that is waiting for your next move, it is the present that reminds us why we are here and what matters the most right now.

Having lived through cancer, it is much easier for you to reconnect with the now because you have stood on the edge, and you are intimately familiar with how precious and fragile life truly is. You and I know that any day, it can be taken away, and bringing back that sense of immediacy isn't morbid, but a direct route to bringing ourselves back to the present we treasure.

Exercise: Treasure the moment

Whether you are plagued with worry or fed up with the frustration of everyday life, this clarifying question will help you bring yourself back into the reality of what is most important right now.

When there is too much going on, or you don't know what to do next, ask yourself:

If this was my last day alive, what would I do right now?

The more you appreciate life and your place in it, the less room there is for worry.

PART 4

NEGOTIATE
YOUR WAY THROUGH
CHALLENGES

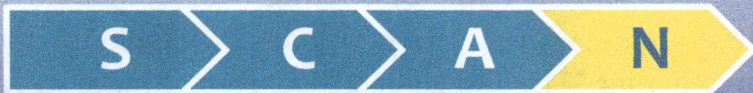

S > C > A > N

On my way to the oncologist's office for my check-up, I kept telling myself—*They would tell the oncologist if there was a problem with one of the tests. Surely, they would find out on the day and he'd let me know ahead of time? There must be an alert of some kind when they find cancer on the CT scan or the blood test. But what if there isn't?* I had never had the courage to ask, an odd superstition, as if by asking I would somehow change the result.

As I walked through the twisting insides of the hospital, I felt my feet getting heavier with every step. I turned into the waiting room. My head blank, hollow, unable to conjure up any thought or image that could distract me from the result. I flicked through a random magazine when Dave, my oncologist, leaned out of his cabinet, "Joe? Come this way!"

With a careful but firm touch he inspects my remaining testicle, and then turns his attention to the lymph nodes in my chest, neck, and abdominal area. With the physical exam over, Dave walks back to his desk to go over the scan reports.

Will I be coming home or coming back to the ward? The seconds of waiting turn into hours. Dave looks up from the computer. "The news is good, Joe, everything is still as we expect it." I breathe a quiet sigh of relief. *Expect? Hope, more like!* I cannot hide the smile that takes over my entire being. "Thank you, Dave, this is the best news I could have hoped for!"

Dave smiles before turning serious again. "One thing we have to keep in mind, though. With the steroids you had during treatment, your body composition has changed..." This term was new to me. "Wait, what do you mean when you say my body composition has changed?"

Dave looks up in thought, then said, "You have put on a fair amount of weight, and I think you should do something about it. You were already in the high-risk group for heart disease after chemo, and this might make things very difficult over time."

This was not what I was expecting. *Haven't I been through enough? What else do I have to put myself through now to get in shape? I've tried getting fit and I failed, and that was before cancer, so what do I do now?*

There is one thing I know now—it's a new lease of life. I am here to enjoy every moment I have with my family and make a difference to others who have experienced this struggle. This is just one part of the journey. I can do this, I can figure it out... There must be a way!

Find Your AIM

No, life after cancer isn't always easy. If anything, cancer has taught me that life is filled with surprises, and not all of them are good. But cancer has also taught me that you can get through it. If you can weather the storm, then you look to the future with hope.

When you know there will be obstacles in your way, you can anticipate the challenges and work around them. When you expect challenges and you plan to get through them, you will keep your balance at a time when you need it the most.

Our AIM is to negotiate our way through setbacks and challenges by having a clear process to deal with them when they come up:

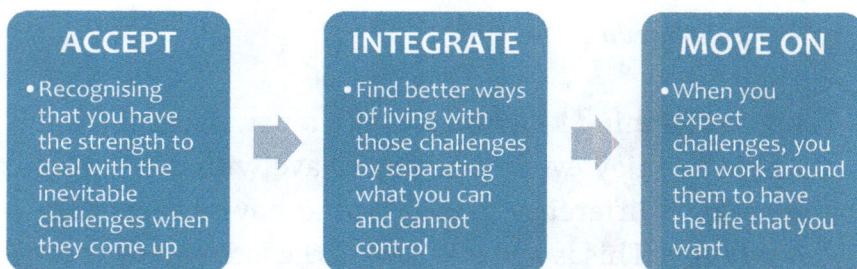

ACCEPT		INTEGRATE		MOVE ON
• Recognising that you have the strength to deal with the inevitable challenges when they come up	→	• Find better ways of living with those challenges by separating what you can and cannot control	→	• When you expect challenges, you can work around them to have the life that you want

We are strong enough to accept challenges as a part of our lives. They do not prevent us from aiming high and living a life of impact, of joy and fulfilment.

When I found out I had to lose weight if I didn't want to risk having my life cut short by heart disease, I chose to accept the challenge. At that point, I had failed at every attempt to eat healthy and cut back on snacks and beer. I had quit gym at least three times. I had been a chain smoker for over ten years. But the change never stuck because I always forced myself into it—this time, change was what I truly WANT.

I found an exercise physiologist who specialises in helping people after cancer, and I stuck to the workout she created for me. I saw a dietician who is familiar with cancer, and we found a plan that fits in with my life and my time with the family. I started exercising three times a week, cut down on late-night snacks, and learned how to make salads.

It wasn't easy, and there were times when I thought about giving up or going easy on myself, but still, I kept going. I knew the challenges would come at some point, so I built up habits in such a way that I could not go around them. With a string of regular reminders popping up in my phone and early-morning routines that did not stop me from going to work on time, I kept showing up, day after day. There wasn't much to show for it in the beginning except sweat, muscle aches, and exhaustion, but slowly, I started seeing results. Kilo after kilo got wiped off the scales, centimetre after centimetre disappeared from my waistline, which gave me the inspiration and confidence to do anything I set my mind to.

✏️ Exercise: Negotiate life around challenges

Start each day by anticipating the obstacles you might face. Use this prompt in your journal:

If there is one challenge I'm ready to face today, it is...

This prompt makes me think of potential challenges, whether it is something I'm not good at, a situation that bothers me, or something that is holding me back. Here are some real-life examples:

- If there is one challenge I'm ready to face today, it is to not lose my temper like I did yesterday.
- If there is one challenge I'm ready to face today, it is the big pitch—bring it on!
- If there is one challenge I'm ready to face today, it is practising my speech for at least one hour.

When you expect the struggle, you are ready to face the day. It may not be easy, but you decide that you are going to show up at your best, and hope that it will be enough.

Cancer has taught us that we are resilient in the face of struggle. It has proven beyond any reasonable doubt that we can survive despite the worry and the changes we never asked for. After surviving cancer, we have come to accept that we will be living with the unknown. But the uncertainty that you might get cancer is a better alternative than the certainty of seeing the scan with the tumours inside you.

You are still here, my friend. You have stopped fighting and started living. You deserve the life you want, and you will prevail, despite the challenges that may come your way!

YOU ALREADY OWN EVERYTHING THAT YOU WILL EVER HAVE

Some say, "I won't let cancer define me." But how can it not? It's an epic experience that is bound to define you in some way. And if it will define you anyway, then you might as well have a say in *how* it does that from now on.

Cancer is the readymade explanation for why you are miserable. Some people are very understanding—after all, you have been through a lot, and no one expects you to live a good life.

They expect that you will never recover, that you come out damaged, shattered, living in the shadow of your disease. It's not what other people might expect that counts, but what they see you do now.

In life, no one will tell you—from now on, you can stop worrying and follow your dreams.

Nobody will say—from this day on, things will turn out the way they should.

No one will take away your sorrows, past hurts, and regrets.

No one will give you the time you need to change your career, go on a big trip to Alaska, or renovate your kitchen.

No one can give you the life you want because you already own everything that you will ever have!

The life where you wake up and look forward to what the day might bring.

The life filled with small things that give you joy.

The life you spend with people who respect you and cherish the time you spend together.

The life where you make a difference that is meaningful to you and aligned with your values, so that you feel like you belong.

This life is already here, and it's waiting for you to take it.

You don't have to wait another second—you decide whether you want to claim it right now!

Because after what you have been through—isn't that enough?

Isn't this a second (or third, or more, if you had a recurrence) chance in life, a new opportunity to make things right?

As you look ahead to scan life for opportunities to make things right, it isn't always easy to find the best way forward—sometimes you'll want someone by your side to help you work through worries, figure out what to do next, and stay on track towards your goals.

Honestly, I wish I had had someone like that after my cancer treatment. That is why I put together a coaching program called *Take Your Life Back After Cancer*. This program has been designed to support you in several ways:

- Live with and accept the changes brought on by cancer
- Tackle worries about cancer coming back
- Build even stronger bonds with the people you care about
- Discover your true calling
- Enjoy life despite the uncertainty
- Find the time and energy you need to contribute in a meaningful way
- and much, much more.

In this program, you'll work with me during twelve one-on-one sessions. Every session has a different theme to improve one key area of your life, where we talk about specific problems you are facing and how to make things work for your personal situation.

I'm here to help you and support you in taking your life back from cancer.

Apply for a free strategy session to see if we are a good fit: http://TakeYourLifeBackAfterCancer.com or email me directly on joe@simplifycancer.com

My friend, today you have another chance at life, to live fully and openly, without looking back.

The past has already been decided for you, but the future is waiting for you to take it, to be as you want it to be, on your terms.

There is nothing in you that is missing, or wrong.

Today, you already own everything that you will ever have. Now, you just have to make good use of it.

So if you can choose how the cancer will define you, what will it be?